HAIRLOSS GUIDE FOR MEN;

A Holistic Approach To Reclaiming Your Hair and Confidence.

With My Secret Natural Home-Made Remedies for Hairloss Unveiled!

Samuel C. Johnson

Table Of Content

HAIRLOSS GUIDE FOR MEN 1

A Holistic Approach To Reclaiming Your Hair and Confidence. 1

With My Secret Natural Home-Made Remedies for Hairloss Unveiled!...1

Samuel C. Johnson........1

ALOPECIA (HAIRLOSS) 4

Symptoms 6

When hair loss becomes abnormal 6

Origins..........................7

Causes: genes, stress, lifestyle, change of season... 7

Treatments 8

Solutions to fight hair loss...................9

Stress and Bald Hair; Relationship 25

Types of stress induced baldness? 26

How to Prevent Balding When Stressed? 30

Hair Care.......................31

Types of Hair Care......32

Hair Care Products 35

Chemical Medicine to Grow Bald Hair...........38

Natural Medicine for Bald Hair Growth 43

What natural and home remedy works for alopecia? 43

Peppermint Oil 43

Rosemary Oil 45

How to make rosemary oil 45

Apple vineger 47

How to use it? 47

Almonds oil 48

Coconut oil 49

Olive oil 50

Onion Juice 51

How to use it? 51

Green Tea 52

How to use it? 53

Biotin 54

Aloe vera 55

How to use it? 56

Lavender oil 56

Cayenne flower 58

How to use it? 58

Nettle oil 59

How to use it? 60

Ginger oil 60

How to use? 61

What shampoo is good for alopecia? 62

How do I prepare it?...63

Application mode 64

The important thing about this shampoo for hair loss is that you use it frequently, every other day, or twice a week.........................64

Tips to Reduce Hair Loss 66

My Secret Natural Homemade Remedies to

regain your hair back in a month 70

Instant Hair Growth Oil 71

The Anti Dandruff and Growth Herbal Shampoo 72

Cloves + Rosemary Rinse 73

ALOPECIA (HAIRLOSS)

Alopecia also known as Hairloss is a common thing. In 1 day, normally around 50-100 strands of hair will fall out. If the amount is more than that and continues continuously, you are experiencing severe hair loss and need to get proper treatment to prevent baldness.

Treatment for hair loss itself is very diverse. Before using hair growth drugs, laser therapy, or hair transplant procedures, there's no harm in trying various natural ways to deal with hair loss that are easy to do at home.

When you have alopecia or start losing a lot of hair, it is essential that you treat the problem quickly. Alopecia in men, which is normally hereditary, can be stopped thanks to specific anti-hair loss treatments, which I would be sharing with you in this book. It is also important to avoid stress and eat balanced.

Symptoms

When hair loss becomes abnormal
We all lose between 50 and 80 hairs a day. Like our skin cells, our hair renews itself naturally. New hairs with an average life cycle of 2 to 7 years replace those we lose daily. And each hair follicle produces a new shaft during its growth phase. Our hair can experience between 25 and 30

cycles throughout our entire life. However, when combined with other factors, the hair loss process can accelerate. When there are no new stems to replace the hair we lose, the hair becomes lighter in several areas.

Origins

Causes: genes, stress, lifestyle, change of season...
For men, hair loss is mainly due to genetics. In fact, hereditary androgenetic alopecia affects approximately 70% of men and is caused by an excess of male hormones, androgens. More commonly known as male pattern baldness, androgenetic alopecia can manifest at a

very young age, around 18 years of age.

Progressively, hair growth slows and the cycle is reduced to one year instead of three or four. The hair follicle is less embedded in the dermis and begins to atrophy.

Consequence: hair becomes finer. The hairline on the scalp begins to recede at the temples, forehead and on the top of the head.

Hair loss can be caused by:
- medicines, such as blood thinners or cancer treatments
- a psychological shock
- stress
- unbalanced diets, etc.
- seasonal change
- Lifestyle

Treatments

Solutions to fight hair loss

Before we start to give home remedies for hairloss, we recommend that you daily:

- Use mild shampoos and avoid products that are aggressive to your hair.
- rest and avoid stress
- eat in a healthy and balanced way

This is a natural way to deal with hair loss

Even though it seems simple, home treatments can help overcome hair loss, and even stimulate hair growth. The following are some natural ways to deal with hair loss that you can try:

1. Don't wash your hair too often

Many people think that washing your hair every day can keep your hair healthy. However, this is not entirely true. Washing your hair using shampoo too often can actually cause your hair to become damaged, dry, break easily and look thinner.

Especially if you dry your hair by rubbing your hair with a towel. Therefore, it is recommended that you only wash your hair 1-3 times a week. Next, dry your hair by gently patting the towel on your hair.

2. Style your hair gently

Various hair styling methods, such as coloring,

straightening and curling hair, can make hair damaged and dry and irritate the scalp. Meanwhile, the habit of tying and braiding hair too tightly can also cause hair roots to be pulled, so that hair falls out easily.

In order to minimize hair loss and keep your scalp healthy, you should avoid the hair styling mentioned above. If you want to dry your hair with a hair dryer, avoid using hot temperatures because it can damage your hair quickly.

3. Adopt a healthy lifestyle

Several types of diseases, such as malnutrition and anemia or lack of blood, can cause hair loss . Therefore, to prevent and treat hair loss, try to live a healthy lifestyle by eating healthy foods and exercising regularly.

4. Use hair oil

Using hair oil can also reduce hair loss. Therefore, there is no harm in using natural oils, such as coconut oil, to treat your hair loss. Lauric acid, which is found in coconut oil, can help bind proteins in hair. So, it can protect it from damage to the roots and hair strands.

Coconut oil contains healthy fatty acids needed to stimulate new hair growth. To get this benefit, you can apply enough coconut oil to your scalp, then massage gently with circular movements.

Apply the remaining oil on your hands to other parts of your hair, including the ends of your hair. After that, cover it with a towel and leave it overnight, then wash your hair until clean.

5. Use a hair mask

Regularly using a hair mask can not only make hair more moist, but can also reduce hair loss. You can make a mask for hair loss yourself at home using natural ingredients, such as egg yolk and aloe vera.

Egg yolk contains vitamin A, biotin, amino acids and folate which can increase hair growth. Meanwhile, aloe vera contains vitamin C, vitamin E, vitamin B12, folic acid and choline which are useful for strengthening hair.

6. Get enough hair nutrition

Not only from the outside, you also have to care for your hair from the inside by eating nutritious food so that hair loss can be reduced. Some of the nutrients needed to treat hair loss include vitamin A and zinc.

Vitamin A is needed to stimulate hair growth, so that hair does not become thin. Zinc is no different. This nutrient is also needed to stimulate growth and repair hair tissue and maintain hair's natural moisture. Apart from that, the addition of argan cream and avocado essence from the outside can help maintain natural shine and strengthen hair, so hair remains healthy.

7. Massage the Scalp

Maybe if you go to a salon they will definitely offered a scalp massage, and it feels good, right? Can it help grow hair too? Possible.

8. Do the Mediterranean Diet

The Mediterranean diet is a diet that involves consuming foods containing raw vegetables and fresh herbs. It has been revealed that a diet containing raw vegetables and fresh herbs can reduce the risk of androgenic alopecia.

To get the best results, a person needs to consume high amounts of this diet food. For example, consume parsley, basil, green salad more than three days a week.

9. Use Olive Oil

Hair loss treatment can use olive oil, to protect hair from dryness or other hair damage. Olive oil is also the main ingredient for implementing the Mediterranean diet to condition hair.

In this way, the benefit of olive oil for hair is that it can help slow down genetic hair loss. You can apply a few tablespoons of olive oil directly to your hair, then let it sit for 30 minutes before washing your hair.

10. Consume Protein

Hair follicles are mostly made of protein, called keratin. A 2017 study by Dinesh Gowda, et al, from Hairline International Hair Clinic India, recorded 100 people with hair loss known to be caused by nutritional deficiencies.

Hair nutrition includes amino acids, which function as building blocks for protein. Researchers Emily L Guo from Baylor College of Medicine and Rajani Katta from Houston Methodist

Hospital USA, found that eating foods rich in protein can help prevent hair loss. Foods that are rich in protein include eggs, nuts, fish, low-fat dairy products, chicken, and many more.

11. Multivitamin Supplements

Hind M. Almohanna, et al, from Dermatology and Therapy in their research published in 2018 stated that vitamins A, B, C, D, iron, selenium and zinc are important in helping the hair growth and retention process. You can find a daily multivitamin at most drug stores or ask your doctor to prescribe one. Vitamin A consists of retinoids, which can increase hair growth. Vitamin A also helps sebum production, which can keep the scalp healthier.

Joyce Hoot, et al, from the University of Pittsburgh, in a journal published by the National Library of Medicine in 2018, noted that vitamin D is associated with alopecia. Vitamin D helps treat deficiencies, which can help hair regrowth.

12. Consume Biotin

Biotin (vitamin H) or B7 plays a role in the synthesis of fatty acids in the body, which in the process is an important part of the hair life cycle. People who are deficient in biotin may experience hair loss.

You can take 3-5 milligrams of biotin every day, to treat hair loss. But, for further information, you need to discuss with your doctor about the best way to consume biotin

13. Ginseng Supplements

Ginseng can help increase
hair growth on the scalp,
because it contains certain
phytochemicals. This is what
was written in research by Bu
Young Choi from Seowon
University, in the
International Journal of
Molecular Sciences, published
in 2018.

However, there needs to be
further study to recommend a
certain dose for using it. To
take ginseng supplements,
you need to talk to your
doctor about topical solutions
that contain this ingredient.

14. Onion Juice

Onion juice helps grow hair
for people with alopecia
areata. You can treat hair loss

naturally by applying raw onion juice to your scalp twice a day.

While research on this treatment is limited, onion juice appears to increase growth by nearly 87%. Khalifa E. Sharquie and Hala K. Al-Obaidi in the Japanese Dermatological Association journal published in 2014, scientists believe the magic lies in the onion content.

15. Yoga

Hair loss is also caused by stress. This is related to telogen effluvium (TE) which occurs when there is a change in the number of hair follicles. If these changes occur during the telogen phase, they can cause hair loss.

Yoga may help with this. Try doing yoga poses to relieve

stress, to prevent and slow hair loss.

The yoga poses that can be done include dog facing the crater, forward bend, camel pose, kneeling pose and many more. You can easily find free yoga poses on YouTube too, you know.

16. Use essential oils

The way to treat excessive hair loss with natural ingredients is using essential oils. A 1998 study conducted by IC Hay, et al, from the Department of Dermatology, Aberdeen Royal Infirmary divided 86 people with alopecia areata into two groups.

The study tried mixing essential oil (cedarwood) with lavender and rosemary onto their scalps. After 7 months, 43% of the group showed improvement in the condition of their hair.

Androgenetic alopecia is the most common among the male population—it affects up to 80% of men at some point in their lives—although women also suffer from it, especially after the age of 70. The causes are genetic and hormonal, since androgens are largely responsible for a miniaturization of hair that can lead to hair loss.

Have you noticed the first symptoms of androgenic alopecia? Are you wondering what can I apply for hair loss? The most common first step is to look for natural remedies to delay its progression and stop hair loss. Although it is recommended that a specialist diagnose what type of alopecia you suffer from in order to face it with the most appropriate treatment, there are home remedies for hair loss that can be helpful.

These are some:

- Rosemary.
- Apple vinager.
- Almonds oil.
- Coconut oil.
- Olive oil.
- Onion.
- Green Tea.
- Biotin.
- Vitamins.

To improve our general health and, therefore, strengthen our hair, it is highly recommended to quit smoking , since it has been proven that it increases the risk of suffering from androgenic alopecia. Reducing stress is also important.

Stress and Bald Hair; Relationship

Hair loss is something that is worrying, especially if the loss that occurs causes you to experience baldness. Well, many people suspect that stress can inhibit hair growth, so you can experience baldness. How can stress make your hair bald? The following is a complete explanation.

Psychosocial stress is reported to have an important role in the occurrence of baldness. According to one study, the number of patients with baldness triggered by stress was recorded at 6.7 to 96 percent. Well, psychosocial stress itself occurs when you feel a threat from your own social environment, for example when you feel very pressured by the success of your colleagues in the office, so that you become inferior and down or when you feel abandoned by friends who often go out with you without inviting you.

This type of stress usually has a big impact on health. The reason is, psychosocial stress makes sufferers feel isolated, lonely and without support. One of the impacts on health is that it causes hair to go bald due to loss.

Types of stress induced baldness?

There are three types of baldness that can be caused

by excessive stress. For further information about the three types of baldness, please see the information below.

1. **Alopecia Areata**

Alopecia areata (baldness) is an inflammatory process or autoimmune disease that occurs with hair loss. Many factors influence baldness, including autoimmune, genetic, emotional and environmental diseases. Alopecia areata attacks the scalp, but areas of the body covered with hair can also be affected by this problem. The hair loss that occurs usually has a circular pattern and is progressive, and can also cause baldness throughout the entire head area (alopecia totalis). Although the cause is still unclear, several studies suggest a link between stress and alopecia areata .

2. **Telogen Effluvium**

One of the most common causes of stress causing hair loss is through telogen effluvium . Normally, you will lose about a hundred strands of hair a day, but stress can cause you to lose more hair than necessary. Well, unnatural hair loss is also called telogen effluvium .

Your hair normally grows in a cycle. In the active phase, hair grows over several years. After the active phase, your hair enters the resting phase. This resting phase lasts approximately three months after your hair falls out. On average, normal hair loss is around 100 hairs per day. The hair will then be replaced within six months by new hair.

When your body is under stress or you feel negative emotional turmoil, hair will fall out more easily. When stressed, most of your hair will enter the resting phase before it's time. Furthermore, the hair will fall out three months later.

3. **Trichotillomania**

Trichotillomania is a habit caused by stress and anxiety when someone pulls their hair without realizing it. This can damage hair and cause baldness because it is pulled too often.

How to Prevent Balding When Stressed?

Simple lifestyle changes can help reduce baldness, for example by getting enough sleep (approximately 7 hours), drinking lots of mineral water, and consuming foods rich in protein.

Nutrition is important for hair growth. The relationship between food and hair is very close. Hair is made of a protein called keratin. So, you should increase your protein intake.

Lack of protein consumption forces your body to store existing protein for other purposes, such as forming cells. It is believed that spinach, nuts, tofu and milk are good foods for healthy hair. Green tea is also good for inhibiting Dihydrotestosterone (DHT), a hormone that causes hair loss.

Hair Care

Hair care is an overall term for the cleanliness and grooming of the hair that grows on the human scalp. Apart from making hair shiny, hair care also has the function of making hair healthy and smooth and free from hair loss and dandruff. Hair treatments are usually done in salons, and some are traditionally done at home.

In ancient times, Egyptian women used animal fat to

style their hair. Women in Europe use roots, flowers and jewelry to decorate their hair. Apart from that, sometimes to care for their hair they often use vinegar and fermented liquids and leeches to protect their hair from the heat of the sun.

Types of Hair Care

1. Keratin Treatment

Keratin is a protein that can be found in hair, skin and nails. About 95% of keratin is found in the hair. Keratin functions to protect the outer layer of each hair strand, and provides strength from within the hair. Hair treatment using keratin techniques is usually done to straighten hair. As a result, it can straighten hair for three months. The keratin hair treatment technique is done by applying keratin cream to the hair, starting from the roots to the hair shaft, then leaving it for 30 minutes, until the keratin absorbs the scalp and hair, after which the hair is washed and straightened.

2. Scalp Scrub

Scrubs are fine granules that are rubbed on the skin, which function to remove dead skin cells. The goal is to soften and smoothen the skin. Giving a scrub to the scalp aims to remove dead skin cells and dirt on the scalp. Applying a scrub to the skin is done in the same way as using shampoo, by wetting the hair before applying the scrub to the hair. The final process is washing the hair.

3. **Creambath**

Creambath is a type of hair and scalp treatment by applying special cream to the head. The cream provided is the result of a mixture of chemicals and natural ingredient extracts. The function of the cream used is to maintain the moist quality of the hair, prevent hair from breaking, and strengthen the hair shaft so it doesn't split.

4. **Hot Oil Treatment**

Giving therapy with hot oil on the head makes the body relax. For hair, applying hot oil is useful for improving blood circulation, preventing dandruff from the scalp, and protecting hair from weather changes. How to care for hair using this technique, starting from heating the oil, with the help of hot water or a small stove. The oil chosen is coconut oil which is useful for providing nutrition to the hair. Castor oil is useful for making hair fertile. Almond oil is useful for nourishing hair, and olive oil is useful for caring for hair and scalp.

Hair Care Products

1. Shampoo

Shampoo is a term that originates from Indian colonialism. In ancient times, when carrying out head massage activities, colonialists usually used oil. In the 19th century, the use of soap began to appear to clean hair. However, soap is not suitable for hair. This is because soap can cause scalp irritation and result in a thin layer on the hair and dullness.

Hair requires an acidic pH of around 4-5, while soap has an alkaline pH of around 8.5. Shampoo is a hair care product that is the basis of cosmetic hair care treatments. Shampoo comes in thick liquid form, also in bar form. Shampoo can replace soap to clean the scalp, the difference being that shampoo is responsible for removing dandruff, environmental dust and residue from hair care products.

2. Softeners (Conditioners)

Softeners or conditioners are additives that function to soften hair. Hair softeners appeared following technological developments, this is because shampoo can only remove sebum. Hair requires substances such as synthetic sebum or conditioner which can increase hair shine, volume and improve hair manageability, as well as maintain hair styling.

Chemical Medicine to Grow Bald Hair

The following are several types of medicine for hair growth for frontal baldness that have been determined by the Indonesian Association of Skin and Venereology Specialists.

1. Minoxidil (Rogaine)

Minoxidil is a hair growth drug that can be purchased at the pharmacy. This medicine is in liquid form and some are in foam form. Minoxidil is able to widen the blood vessels in the scalp, so that the hair follicles get optimal nutrition and oxygen. This way of working stimulates hair growth.

This hair loss medicine is used by rubbing it on the scalp twice every day. Use no more than 2 ml per day. At least, it takes 6 months to get new, stronger hair. The reason is, at the beginning of using this drug, the hair that grows can be very thinner than the previous hair.

Although it can help grow hair, minoxidil has side effects such as scalp irritation, unwanted hair growth on the skin of the face or on the hands, and a faster heart rate (tachycardia). Please remember, this drug is classified as strong, so a doctor's prescription must be used.

2. Finasteride (Propecia)

This is a male hair grower that is available in the form of oral medication. Women should not take this medicine. Apart from helping hair grow, this drug reduces hair loss. The dose of this hair growth drug is given at 1 mg once a day.

Finasteride is also usually combined with topical minoxidil . Side effects of finasteride include reduced sexual drive, depression, and increased risk of prostate cancer. However, this side effect of cancer is very rare. This medicine is also classified as strong, so you need to buy it with a doctor's prescription.

3. Dutasteride

Dutasteride is one of the strong oral medications that a

doctor may prescribe to grow hair. This drug works by inhibiting the hormone that causes male baldness, namely dihydrosterone or DHT. Doctors usually give a dose of 0.5 mg once a day.

Keep in mind, this is a men's hair grower. Women should not consume it and can only get it with a doctor's prescription. The side effects of the drug that you may experience are reduced libido, impotence, and difficulty ejaculating.

Natural Medicine for Bald Hair Growth

What natural and home remedy works for alopecia?

Here are several types of natural remedies for bald hair growth that you can try at home. We recommend that you try some of these natural remedies against hair loss to see which one works best for you. They are easy to find ingredients that you can include in your routine with very little effort:

Peppermint Oil

A study published by Toxicological Research (2014)

found that peppermint oil can increase hair growth more effectively than jojoba oil, and minoxidil, which is often used to treat hair loss.

Researchers also found that hair treatment with this oil can increase scalp thickness and the number of hair follicles. Peppermint oil for hair contains menthol which causes the blood vessels just under the scalp to dilate. This additional blood flow can help promote further hair growth. It is not surprising that peppermint oil can be used as a hair growth essential oil.

Rosemary Oil

The benefits of rosemary for hair are multiple, but the main advantage is its vasodilating effect, which promotes blood circulation to the follicles. This way they receive more nutrients, so the hair remains strong. It can be applied in the form of rosemary oil, with a gentle massage. It is also anti-inflammatory, so it calms and balances irritated scalps .

How to make rosemary oil

- Wash the rosemary branches well and let them dry completely.
- Place the rosemary in a container without removing any part, since

everything in this plant
is usable.

- Then, completely cover
the rosemary with olive
oil and cover the
receptacle.
- The next step is to leave
the container with the
oil and rosemary in
a warm, dark place to
marinate and rest for at
least a month.
- Finally, after this
time, strain the oil and
place it in a glass jar .
- With these simple
guidelines you will
obtain a 100% natural,
ecological and artisan
rosemary oil so you can
enjoy its multiple
benefits

Apple vineger

Apple cider vinegar or simply apple cider vinegar is nothing more than fermented juice. Helps keep the pH of the scalp balanced. In addition, it is useful to prevent frizz and soften hair, which will appear thicker and shinier.

As a home treatment for hair loss in women and men, it is believed to prevent hair loss by promoting blood flow to the scalp. In turn, it can soften the hair and its pH helps eliminate fungi, bacteria and restore the acidity of the skin.

How to use it?
Dilute a little apple cider vinegar in warm water.

Then, use it after washing on a
very small area of the scalp
and let it sit for 10 minutes to
see if you have any allergies.

If you don't find anything
unusual, you can apply it all
over your scalp and hair.

Leave it on for 5 minutes and
rinse with plenty of water.

Use it once a week, always
diluted in warm water, and
apply it after washing to the
ends and scalp, massaging
gently. Leave it on for a few
minutes and remove with
plenty of water to eliminate
the odor.

Almonds oil

This oil is very easy to find in
herbalists, specialized stores

and even pharmacies. It is rich in vitamin E, a natural antioxidant that is very beneficial for skin and hair. Applying it is simple: place a few drops on the scalp and massage gently, if possible daily. This way you will be able to nourish the hair fibers, hydrate them and recover damaged hair, in addition to providing shine and softness.

Coconut oil

Another option to prevent hair loss is to massage your head after washing and for a few minutes with coconut oil. Leave it on for half an hour, so that the fatty acids that make it up penetrate the cuticle and strengthen its structure. Coconut also restores balance to the scalp's pH . It contains vitamin E, key to strengthening hair fibers, and has antimicrobial, antibacterial and antifungal properties. Without a doubt, it is a natural remedy against alopecia that should be taken into account.

Olive oil

We just have to apply a few drops of extra virgin olive oil to our hair and massage gently for fifteen minutes to benefit from its properties. Its high content of vitamin E and K helps repair and strengthen hair, making it less brittle. In addition, it protects it from external aggressions, especially the sun, while

hydrating and nourishing it,
and repairing the scalp.

Onion Juice

Hair juice is also a well-
known home remedy against
alopecia, because it stimulates
circulation, increases blood
flow that feeds the follicle and
enhances hair regeneration.

How to use it?
To perform this home
treatment for hair loss in men,
peel 4 medium onions and cut
them into small pieces.

Then, extract their juice by
squeezing them with the same
blade you cut them with or
with a juicer.

Next, apply the juice to a
small area of the skin and wait

until the next day to find out if it causes any type of allergy in you.

If you don't see anything strange, you can apply it to the roots of your hair twice a day for 8 weeks. You can leave this onion mask on for 20 minutes before rinsing it off.

Another way will be;

To apply it to the hair, you can also grind it until you get a paste, which we will then strain to obtain the juice. Diluted in water or essential oil, just leave it on your hair for a few minutes before shampooing.

Green Tea

It is well known that tea contains a large amount of antioxidants, which are essential to enhance hair growth, as well as its strengthening. In addition, it is rich in minerals such as sodium, magnesium, potassium and iron.

Drinking green tea can be good for your health. But, did you know that its topical application can also have benefits for your hair? In this sense, there are various studies that have investigated its properties. Its action seems to be due to components such as catechins, which help control hair loss and promote growth.

How to use it?

Make an infusion with 150 milliliters of hot water and 5 grams of green tea.

Then, once it's cool, pour very little onto a small area of your head. Wait about 30 minutes to see if you have any unwanted effects.

If not, carefully pour it all over your hair. You can use it as a toner after washing.

Biotin

Biotin for hair is also a well-known ally, key in the formation of hair. It helps strengthen hair, preventing it from becoming brittle, and improves the condition of the follicles. It is included in the formulation of some hair products to regulate oil and dandruff.

You can easily add it to your diet through foods such as eggs, nuts, salmon, tuna, sardines, peas, bananas and strawberries.

Aloe vera

As popular as the others, aloe vera is frequently recommended to reverse hair loss episodes. Although there is little evidence to support its effects, according to an article in Plant Biotechnology Persa , it can increase blood circulation thanks to the iron it contains.

In any case, you have to be careful with its use. In this sense, adverse effects have been reported after topical application, such as irritation and hives, so these should be taken into account.

How to use it?

Before applying it all over your head, try it on a small area to see if you have a reaction.

If no unwanted effects occur, apply pure aloe vera gel to your scalp once a day. You can rinse it after a few minutes.

Another way to incorporate it, and safer, is through a shampoo that already has it in its composition.

Lavender oil

Another oil popular as one of the remedies for hair loss is lavender oil. Thus, it can be useful to treat alopecia areata. In this sense, it can reduce hair loss in one month and promote growth after 4 weeks. However, its evidence is scarce, so you should use it with caution.

How to use?

To start, take a few drops of lavender essential oil and massage a small area of your scalp with it. See if you experience any reaction after 30 minutes.

If you do not feel irritation, burning or see redness, you can apply it with massages all over your head.

Leave it on for 20 minutes and then rinse. Use it once a day.

Cayenne flower

Another remedy for excessive hair loss is to use cayenne flower for hair . This plant is abundant in antioxidant compounds, such as flavonoids. Due to its properties, it is used in traditional Chinese medicine to promote hair growth.

How to use it?
Take 7 cayenne flowers and boil them together with 250 milliliters of water.

Then, turn off the heat and let the preparation rest for 10 minutes.

Once cool, use the liquid to rinse a small area of your hair. This way, you will check if there is any allergic reaction.

If you don't notice anything strange after 30 minutes, rinse the rest of your head with the preparation. Let it sit for half an hour and rinse.

Nettle oil

It is common to find hair loss products that contain nettle in their composition. Indeed, nettle is used for hair , for example, to stimulate its growth. Therefore, we suggest using its oil to massage your scalp.

Take a few drops of the oil and perform an allergy test on an area of the scalp.

If you do not notice any unfavorable reaction, take more drops and spread them over your head, massaging for 10 minutes.

Then wash your hair.

Ginger oil

The last of these home remedies for hair loss is ginger oil. As indicated by the Journal of Pharmacognosy and Phytochemistry , applying this plant to the scalp can stimulate follicles and promote better hair quality. Even so, you should be careful

with its use, since it continues
under analysis.

How to use?
Before you begin, perform an
allergy test on a small area of
your scalp. If you don't notice
any unwanted effects, you can
continue.

Then, take a few drops and
massage your entire head for
10 minutes.

Once that time has passed,
rinse.

What shampoo is good for alopecia?

To notice the effects of any anti-hair loss shampoo, the key is consistency in its use, in addition to correct application . It must also be taken into account that it is not a remedy against alopecia in itself, but rather a complement to a treatment prescribed by the specialist or a measure to slow the rate of hair loss

Well, the first thing we are going to need is a natural shampoo with a neutral pH. We are going to use it as a base to include the rest of the elements.

Those normally used for babies are very suitable. They

tend to be the most natural on the market. A small bottle is enough, the standard one you'll find in stores.

- To make our shampoo for hair loss, we will use rosemary essential oil. It has been used for its effects to reactivate blood flow, providing strength to our hair.
- We will also need lemon essential oil . It is a great antiseptic and refreshing.
- We are also going to need two vitamin E capsules . You can find them in natural stores, as well as in pharmacies.

How do I prepare it?

- It's very simple, you just have to pour ten drops of rosemary essential oil and ten drops of lemon essential oil into the neutral shampoo.
- Then, don't forget to add the two vitamin E capsules.
- We shake the shampoo bottle well and we will have it ready.

Application mode

The important thing about this shampoo for hair loss is that you use it frequently, every other day, or twice a week.
You should apply it to damp hair and massage the scalp for at least 10 minutes.

- Then, allow it to act for another 10.
- At the end, rinse with warm water (never hot).

Tips to Reduce Hair Loss

1. Use Phenylephrine

Topical phenylephrine can help treat hair loss, by stimulating the follicle muscles to contract.

2. Avoid touching your hair

There are some people who have a habit of pulling and pulling out their hair. If that's the case, the tip for reducing hair loss is to avoid pulling, twisting or rubbing your hair as much as possible.

3. Dry your hair after shampooing

The easy way to deal with hair loss naturally is always after gently drying your hair with a towel. Avoid rubbing your hair with the towel, and don't twist it in the towel.

4. Choose a Hairstyle

Hairstyles such as braids or tight ponytails can pull hair down to the roots. Well, it turns out that this has the potential to cause excessive hair loss.

John McCoy, et al, in the journal Dermatologic Therapy published in 2017, choosing a hairstyle without overdoing it can avoid irritation to the scalp. Styling your hair with tools that use electric heat, such as curling irons or hair straighteners, can damage or break the hair shaft.

5. Plasma Injection

Injecting platelet-rich plasma (PRP) into the scalp can be a tip to reduce hair loss. This can help stimulate growth in areas already affected by hair loss.

Also Know Some Triggers for Hair Loss

Many factors trigger the rate of hair growth, including:

- Genetics
- Hormonal changes/imbalance
- Malnutrition
- Drugs
- Stress and anxiety
- Disease or other condition

It's best to see a doctor or a health professional to treat unexplained hair loss. So, they

can determine the best way to
deal with excessive hair loss.

So, that's information about
how to treat excessive hair
loss with natural ingredients.
Apart from knowing the
causes of hair loss, you can
also apply the hair care
methods above to prevent hair
loss!

My Secret Natural Homemade Remedies to regain your hair back in a month

Under this section, I will be sharing with you 3 potent recipes that I used when hairloss hit me in my mid twenties, my hairline was receeding and thinning out before my very eyes. Oh! It was one of the scariest moments of my life and trust me when I say, this is now a thing of the past. Not only did my hairline stop receding after discovering and making use of this recipe, but also my hair stopped falling off and my hair became fuller and looked healthy again. I regained my confidence again and honestly, that is my goal; to help you regain your confidence again!

Instant Hair Growth Oil

For this Oil which is my first secret recipe, you would need to get these Ingredients;

- 1 Tsp of Cloves
- 2 Tsp of moringa powder
- 1Tsp of Rosemary
- Coconut Oil
- Jojoba Oil
- Olive Oil

Just add these ingredients together, leave to sit for 2/3 days, Seive and use as a Hair

Oil. Remember, Consistency
is Key!

The Anti Dandruff and Growth Herbal Shampoo

You wouldn't know the efficacy of this shampoo in combination with the above Instant Hair growth oil recipe. To get this shampoo made, you need to get these ingredients:

- 1 Tsp of Black Seed; Help strengthen Hair
- 1Tsp of Fenugreek; Fights Dandruff
- 1 Tsp of StarAnise; Treats Itchy scalp
- 1Tsp of Hibiscus; Treats flaky scalp and dandruff

- 1Tsp of Rosemary; For Hair Growth.

Mix all dry ingredients together and pour hot water over it, allow to sit for 50min to 1 hour.

Strain and add 1 cup of Castile Soap – Castile soap is a clear liquid soap base made from olive oil and does not contain animal fat and very vegan friendly.

Use as a Shampoo.

Shelf life ; ¾ weeks. Just keep in a cool dry place.

Cloves + Rosemary Rinse

This recipe is best used right after shampooing and

conditioning your Hair. To get
this Hair Rinse made, you
need to get these ingredients:

- 1Tsp of Cloves
- 1Tsp of Rosemary

Mix the two ingredients inside
a pot or kettle and bring to a
boil for 30 minutes. Drain the
water and allow it cool down.
Store in a container.

It is best used after
shampooing and conditioning
you hair, Just rinse your hair
with it after shampooing and
conditioning.

WARNING:

- If you are allergic to any
  of these ingredients,
  Consult your doctor
  first.

- Do not use Rosemary water/oil if you are hypertensive or allergic.
- Keep Rosemary Water in the fridge and should be used in at least 2 weeks
- Do a patch test first to be sure you are not allergic.

I look forward to you feedbacks on how you've gained your confidence back with your rapid hair growth.

Cheers!